Content

Introduction

01- Be Aware of Virus Around You
02- HPV Causes Genital Infection
03- HPV Causes Cervical Cancer
04- Cancer Targets on Three Men's Organs
05- Penile Cancer on Men
06- The Prostate Cancer on Men: Cause and Effect
07- Effect of HPV on Prostate Cancer
08- Treatment for Prostate Cancer
09- Where is Starting Point of Testicular Cancer?
10- HPV Infects Nasal Cavity
11- Much More Americans Got Oral Infection by HPV Virus
12- Vaccine for Type 16 and 18 Viruses
13- Oral Cancer and HPV
14- HPV types 33 and 45
15- Anal Cancers and HPV
16- Identification of Microorganism in Healthcare
17- Important of Microorganisms in Food Industry
18- Virus that Kill Cancer
19- Perplexing between HIV and HPV

About the Author

 # Cover picture credit for Brandon Brown et al, 2013

Introduction

The title of book: HPV: The Virus Which Donald Trump didn't Know is reflecting to current event where USA president confuses the different between HIV and HPV. Both are viruses that relate human diseases.

HIV responsible for Acquired Immune Deficiency Syndrome (AIDS), while HPV contributes to just annoying diseases to many deadly human cancers. 70 million people infected by HIV and this Virus killed 35 million yearly worldwide.

Hundred million people infected by Human papillomavirus (HPV) globally. 80 million Americans get infected, and more than 30 million new infection each year. HPV is increasingly becoming both global and American problems currently and near future.

This book contains 19 articles which partly from my bloggers. The articles are simple to follow without knowledge of microbiology or health science. By reading the book, at least you will aware about virus, HPV and the different between HPV and HIV.

01- Be Aware of Virus Around You

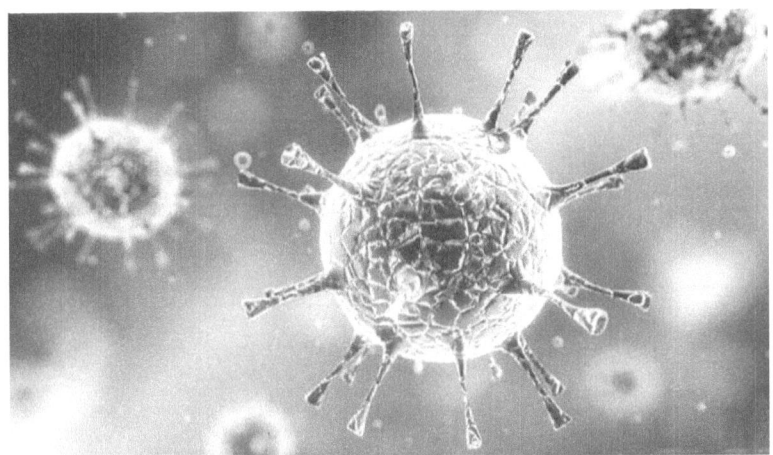

Illustration (m.dailyhunt.in)

HPV stand for Human Papillomavirus, the common virus may associate with human population either in developing or developed countries. Parts of the human body surface, include skin, penis, vagina, anus, vulva and cervix are convenience place to live for HPV. The HPVs may also grow well inside throat and mouth.

It is estimated that approximate 80 million infected by the HPV in the USA, and about 14 million more American infected by HPV each year.

We have identified 100 types or more of HPV, and the number of types could be increasing because identification works are still on going. Many of them present unnoticedly in human body, however, there are dozens of them cause to human diseases. Certain types of virus lead to cancer and serious diseases in human life.

The following Table presents the type of viruses that causes to human diseases:

HPV Types	Diseases
1, 2, 4	Plantar warts
1, 2, 4, 26, 27, 29, 41, 57	Common warts
3, 10, 27, 28, 41, 49	Flat warts
6, 11, 30, 40-45, 51, 54	Genital warts
16, 18, 31, 33, 35, 39, 45, 51, 52, 56, 58	Cervical cancer
16, 18, 34, 39, 42, 55	Precancerous changes
6, 11, 30	Laryngeal papillomas

Table was modified from eMedTV (2017).

The most dangerous virus types are 16, 18, 31, 33, 45, 52 and 58 which relate to cervix, vagina, vulva and anal cancers. Among the less dangerous are 6 and 11, believed to cause genital warts (well known as condylomas).

Actually, there are around 60 (majority) virus types known to cause warts on skin, especially feet and hands. Luckily, wards on feet and hands could not move to infect genital organs, and the other way around.

In regard to Sexually Transmitted Diseases (STD), about 40 virus types associate with STD. Viruses spread through moist layers around the anus and genitals during sexual contact. 1 of 2 (50%) people may infected by HPV if they have sex experience in their life time.

Reference
eMedTV. 2017. Types of HPV. Retrieved from
    http://hpv.emedtv.com/hpv/types-of-hpv.html

02- HPV Causes Genital Infection

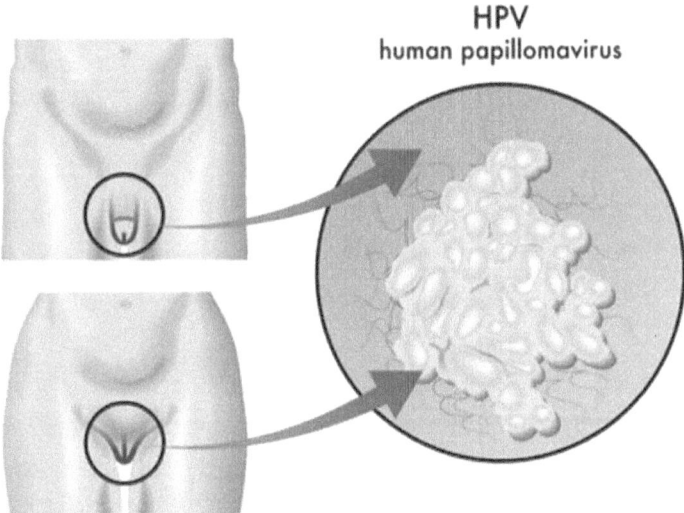

Warts in men and women (https://www.women-info.com)

HPV (Human papillomavirus) that infects human genital may cause range of severity, from just annoying to higher, and even lead to morbidity and mortality.

Warts are common form of the infection in human genitals, caused by HPV type 6 or 11. Even caused 90% genital warts. These types are low risk of viruses. No genital warts are believed to associated to mortality. However, presents of wart could made un-comfortable.

Higher risk viruses such as HPV type 16 and 18 grow into invasive penile cancer in men. These type 16 and 18 known to cause cervices cancer on women as well. Around 70% of cervices cancer cases are caused by these two HPV viruses.

There are around 26 thousand cases of penile cancer in the world every year. As reported by American Cancer Society (2018) that penile cancer is not common in the

USA and Europe compared to other part of the world such as in Asia, Africa, and South America.

The fact so mire for women, there are nearly 300,000 deaths annually due to cervical cancer, and the worse for developing countries with cases of cervical cancer at 80% rate of 300 thousand deaths.

In respect to Sexually Transmitted Infection (STI), HPV is the most common. However, HPV is different compared to deadly virus of HIV (AIDS) and HSV (herpes). It is believed that more than 50% who experienced sex had some types of HPV. Few of virus are dangerous.

Reference

American Cancer Society. (2018). "Key Statistics for Penile Cancer." Retrieved from **Error! Hyperlink reference not valid.** key-statistics.html

03-HPV Causes Cervical Cancer

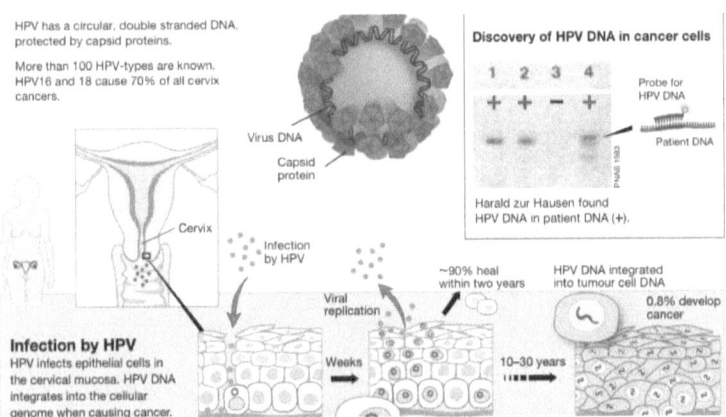

HPV causes cervix cancers
(http://nurseswhovaccinate.blogspot.com)

Human papillomavirus, HPV type 16 and 18 may cause both penile cancer on men and cervices cancer on women as well. Around 70% of cervices cancer cases are caused by these two type of HPV viruses.

Sexual intercourse may expose women genital to HPV. Many women survive from virus infection, but few are vulnerable. Viruses develop slowly, and even convert norm cell on cervix (uterus part which opens to vagina) into cancer cell.

The process from infection into cancel cells takes several years (10 to 30 years). The process could be quicker if infected women are smoking. The same case with penile cancer, where smoking may reduce capability immune system to fight cancer developments.

In the US, there are 12,000 women diagnosed with cervical cancer every year, and 4,000 death every year. The number is estimated will increase in coming years.

Survival rates are depending on several factors, they include race and stage of cancer diagnosed. American Society of Clinical Oncology (ASCO, 2017) reported that

69% and 57% of 5-year survival rate for white and black women consecutively. At early stage of diagnosed, the survival rate may reach 91%.

Reference
American Society of Clinical Oncology (ASCO). 2017.
     Cervical Cancer: Statistics. Retrieved from
     https://www.cancer.net/cancer-types/cervical-cancer/statistics

04-Cancer Targets on Three Men's Organs

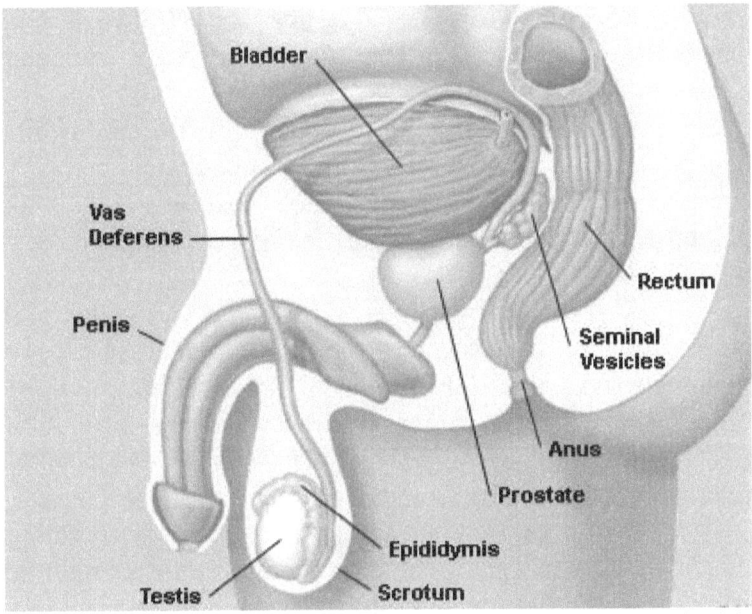

Testis, prostate and penis of male (https://urology.ucsf.edu)

Cancer "targets" on three important men organs, they are penile, prostate and testicular. Hundred thousand of men were diagnosed with these three cancers, and thousands of them died each year in several countries such as UK and US.

The number of men died due to prostate cancer even higher than women died of breast cancer. It is estimated that 26,730 deaths from prostate cancer in the US, and 11,819 men died in the UK every year or equal to every around 45 minutes, there be 1 men death.

Penile cancer mainly on men over 60 years old. Those who diagnosed with penile cancer around 75% above 60, and small percentage only below 50 years old. The survival rate could be higher if the cancer was diagnosed at early stage.

Contrary to prostate and penile cancers, testicular cancer mainly diagnosed to the men at younger ages, between 15 to 45 years old. Average age is 33 years old. There are around 8,850 men diagnosed with testicular cancer in the US.

Most men worry with testicular, prostate and penile cancers. It is because these diseases could change patient's lifestyle and psycho. Other impacts that associate with genital relate cancers are impotence, decreased libido and incontinence.

As reported by Stotts (2004) that testicular and penile cancers are very rare, could be treated and have higher survival rate. Unfortunately, "Prostate cancer, on the other hand, is quite common, difficult to screen, difficult to treat without major sexual problems, and yet receives relatively little funding from the NIH."

Finally, the way to avoid these cancers is by doing diagnosed as early as possible. Prevention efforts could be done easily by not consume tobacco, but to consume low fat and a high fiber diet. Healthy promotion such as doing exercise and maintaining a normal weight is important too.

Reference
Stotts, RC. (2004). Cancers of the prostate, penis, and testicles: epidemiology, prevention, and treatment. Nurs Clin North Am. 2004 Jun;39(2):327-40.

05- Penile Cancer on Men

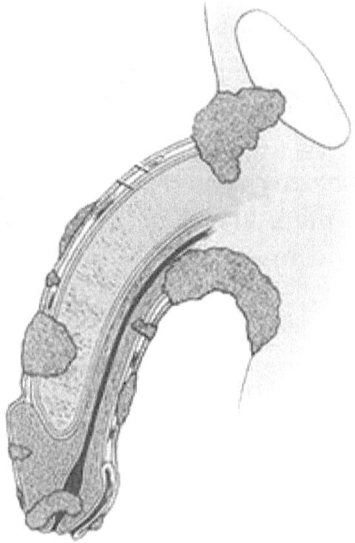

Penile cancer (http://www.medstorerx.com)

High risk HPV virus associates with genital diseases such as "penile cancer" may lead to morbidity and mortality. HPV type 16 and 18 grow or infected in or on the skin of penis, then develop into cancer, called as penile cancer.

Penis skin cell is where almost all penile cancer starts to grow. In specific manner that penis has tissues, the tissues have cell, then penile cancer develops in the cells (different type of cells grows out of control)

One in 100 thousand men diagnosed with penile cancer or 20 thousand cases in the US. There are 500 cases of penile cancer annually in the United Kingdom. Other countries with higher incidence of penile cancer are Denmark and Australia. Unfortunately, there are much more common of penile cancer in developing countries.

Risk of penile cancer may be increased by some factors, include not being circumcised (neonatal circumcision), smoking and poor hygiene. It is understandable relationship between penis cancer and circumcision, or cancer with hygienist.

Question mark is why smoke stimulate penis cancer? The answer is smoking induce immune deficiency, then HPV could attack DNA cell in the penis, thus could increase chance to get penile cancer.

As suggested by Canadian Cancer Society (2018) that "Researchers think that the chemicals in tobacco that cause cancer may damage the DNA in cells of the penis and increase the risk of developing cancer. The risk for cancer may also be higher because smoking increases the risk of an HPV infection not going away."

Combine with human immunodeficiency virus (HIV) infection, smoking men much more vulnerable to immune deficiency, thus immune system will not able to fight penile cancer, even at early stages of cancer developments. Unfortunate for smoking's and AIDS's men, and smoking men with AIDS diseases.

Reference

Canadian Cancer Society. (2018). "Risk factors for penile cancer." Retrieved from http://www.cancer.ca/en/cancer-information/cancer-type/penile/risks/?region=bc#Tobacco

06- The Prostate Cancer on Men: Cause and Effect

PROSTATE CANCER

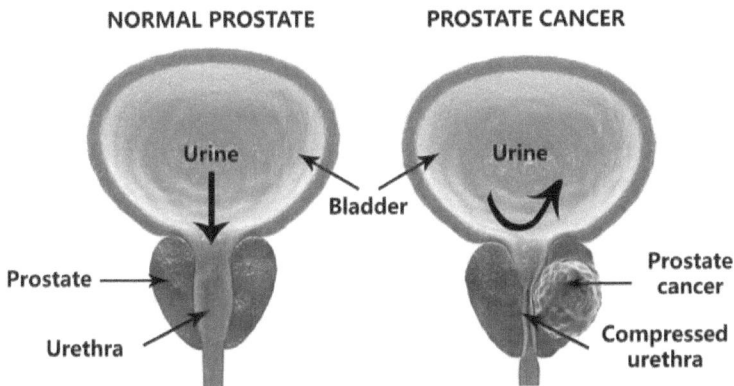

Prostate Cancer (https://www.news-medical.net)

Prostate is the male sex gland responsible for production of fluid that forms part of semen. It surrounds the urethra (the tube that carries urine and semen through the penis and out of the body). Prostate cancer is diseases that effect on men only. Cancer begins in tissues of the prostate gland which is located just below the bladder and in front of the rectum. After skin cancer, prostate cancer is the most common cancer in men in the USA. It is the second leading cause of death from cancer in men.

There are around 209 thousand men were diagnosed, and about 27 thousand dies due to prostate cancer in the USA each year, behind only lung cancer. Reported by the American Cancer Society (2016) that risk of prostate cancer is 1 man in 7 (14.29%) will be diagnosed with prostate cancer during his lifetime. The chance to get cancer will be higher to older men, especially in men of 65 years or older.

From genetic view point, prostate cancer is highly heritable; the inherited risk of prostate cancer has been estimated to be as high as 60%. Men diagnosed with prostate cancer are highly probably coming from close relative (a father or a brother) with prostate cancers. The Memorial Sloan Kettering Cancer Center (2016) suggested that a man with one close relative with prostate cancer is twice as likely to develop cancer, then, If two close male relatives are affected, the risk of developing prostate cancer is increased five-fold compared to man with no family members diagnosed.

There are several hundred genes implicate to different stages of Prostate Cancer. Maqungo et al, (2011) informed that South African National Bioinformatics Institute, University of the Western Cape has developed database called as Dragon Database of Genes associated with Prostate Cancer (DDPC). Data were collected from sources of around the world. Some of genes connected to prostate cancers are BRCA1, BRCA2, and HOXB13. If these genes have mutated due to un-known reasons, men will have a higher risk of developing prostate cancer and, in some cases, other cancers during their lifetimes.

The BRCA1 and BRCA2 genes are involved in fixing damaged DNA, which helps to maintain the stability of a cell's genetic information, thus without these genes or mutations in these genes impair the cell's ability to fix damaged DNA. As these defects accumulate, they can trigger cells to grow and divide uncontrollably and form a tumor (a cancer). Moreover, HOXB13 gene mutations may result in impairment of the protein's tumor suppressor function, resulting in the uncontrolled cell growth and division that can cause to prostate cancer.

Some believe that diets high in animal fats and milk products may be associated with a higher prostate cancer risk. Lack a diet high in red meat and Vitamin D may raise a person's chances of developing prostate cancer. In case of

Vitamin D, Ware (2016) wrote that hormonally active form of vitamin D called "calcitriol" has ability to reduce cancer progression. On the other hand, (Nordqvist, 2016) said that Vitamin D deficiency would cause cancer development unchecked or cause progression of prostate cancer more rapidly.

A diet low in fat and calories and rich in fruits, vegetables, and whole grains is good for our health. Rodriguez (2016) told that if you have prostate cancer, what you eat may play a role in how your cancer progresses and your dietary choices might even influence whether you ever develop the disease at all. Good nutrition is advantage to fight prostate cancer. Nutrition also play role to support prostate cancer treatment. During cancer treatment, it is more important than ever to eat right and get adequate nutrition. It is because cancer patient need strength through excellent diet.

References

American Cancer Society. 2016. Risk of prostate cancer. Retrieved from http://www.cancer.org/cancer/prostatecancer/detailedguide/prostate-cancer-key-statistics.

Memorial Sloan Kettering Cancer Center. 2016. Inherited Risk for Prostate Cancer. Retrieved from https://www.mskcc.org/cancer-care/risk-assessment-screening/hereditary-genetics/genetic-counseling/inherited-risk-prostate

Maqungo, M., Kaur, M., Kwofie, SK., Radovanovic, A., Schaefer, U., Schmeier, S., Oppon, E., Christoffels, A., and Bajic, VB. 2011. DDPC: Dragon Database of Genes associated with Prostate Cancer. Nucleic Acids Res. 2011 Jan; 39(Database issue): D980–D985. Retrieved fromhttp://www.ncbi.nlm.nih.gov/pmc/articles/PMC3013759/

Nordqvist, C. 2016. Prostate Cancer: Symptoms and Causes. Medical News Today. Retrived from http://www.medicalnewstoday.com /articles/ 150086.php? page=2 #causes_ of_prostate_ cancer

Ware, M. 2016. Vitamin D: Health Benefits, Facts and Research. Medical News Today. Retrived from http://www.medicalnewstoday.com/articles/161618.php

07- Effect of HPV on Prostate Cancer

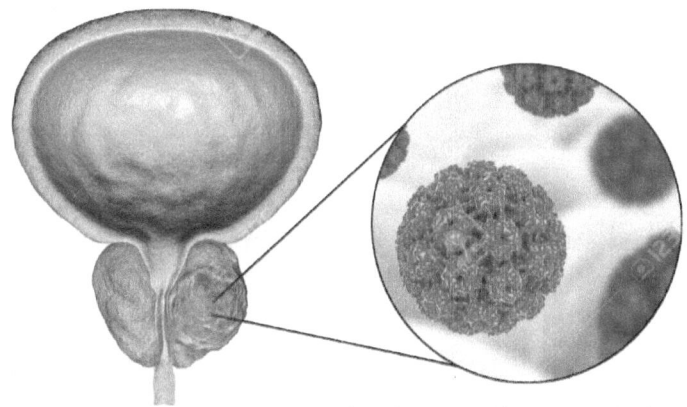

HPV virus infected prostate gland (https://www.123rf.com)

Actually, no clear cut what causes prostate cancer exactly, but some factors may affect the risk. There are many factors that believed to increase the risk to get prostate cancer; some of them are genetics, diet, age, race, lifestyle, obesity and Sexually transmitted diseases (STDs). In this article, we will explore the possibility of prostate cancer caused by HPV virus.

Many researchers believed that there is relationship between HPV infection and prostate cancer (PCa). But, some other scientist doubt about association between HPV and risk of prostate cancer. They have their own arguments and facts either to believe or doubt.

However, study done by Aghakhani (2011) revealed that 74.67% of 150 prostate cancer patients have HPV E7 protein expression. "DNA analysis on a subset of cases confirmed HPV infection and revealed the presence of genotype 16." In term of survival, HPV cancer patients less survive (4.59 years survive) compare to non HPV cancer patient (8.24 years survive).

Other authors, Whitaker et al (2012) found that two viruses, High-risk Human Papilloma Virus and Epstein Barr virus link to cancer development in the prostate gland. More than 50% men with prostate cancer have viruses in their prostate glands. HPV type 18 which is one of high risk viruses found in the prostate samples.

Finally, even some researchers uncertain about HPV virus could cause prostate cancer, it is fact that observations from two different places (Australia and Middle East) indicated strong relationship between HPV and prostate cancer. Moreover, there are abundance of concerning research papers could be searched through Google.

References

Aghakhani, A., Hamkar, R., Parvin, M., Ghavami, N., Nadri,
> M., Pakfetrat, A., Banifazl, M., Eslamifar, A., Izadi N, Jam S., Ramezani, A. (2011). The role of human papillomavirus infection in prostate carcinoma. Scand J Infect Dis. 2011 Jan;43(1):64-9.

Whitaker, NJ., Glenn, WK., Sahrudin, A., Orde, MM.,
> Delprado, W., Lawson, JS. (2012, July 31). "Two viruses link to prostate cancer: High-risk human papilloma virus found with Epstein Barr virus." Retrieved from https://www.sciencedaily.com/releases/2012/07/120731151739.htm

08-Treatment for Prostate Cancer

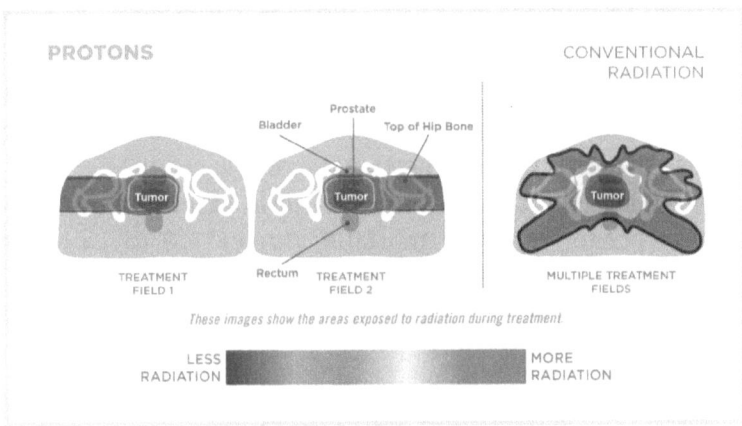

Radiation of prostate cancer
(http://provisionhealthcare.com)

Treatment of prostate cancer depend on the stages whether early or advance stage of cancer. The early stage is indicated by small and localized cancer at prostate gland. Even so small, the cancer can be detected only through a biopsy. At advance stage, cancer looks aggressive more. Cancer may spread outside the prostate to other parts of the body, such as the bones. It is commonly called as metastatic or secondary prostate cancer.

Men when diagnosed at early stage prostate cancer need to wait to be treated. It is because highly likely the cancer will relapse. As explained by Garnick (2016) that men who be cured after treatment for early-stage prostate cancer tend to "biochemical recurrence" or suffer relapse years later. The reason that early stage prostate cancer is too tiny, thus surgeons and radiation oncologists face challenges in eradicating a tumor without causing lasting damage to surrounding organs and structures. Comparable amount of tissue cannot be removed surgically or targeted. Then, these tissues will develop even quicker later on.

The way to cure early stage prostate cancer is explained by Johansson *et al* (2004) that first, wait without initial therapy for certain time, then, do radical local treatment. These procedures will determine the potential for survival benefit following years. Radical treatment called radical prostatectomy reduces prostate cancer mortality by approximately 50%. Moreover, little is known about disease progression and mortality beyond 10 to 15 years after radical treatment.

The advance stage could be called as stage 4 prostate cancers. At this stage the cancers may grow at nearby organs or spreads to other areas of the body. As described by Mayo Clinic Staff (2016) that treatments may slow or shrink an advanced prostate cancer, but for most men, stage 4 prostate cancer isn't curable. Still, treatments can extend the life and reduce the signs and symptoms of cancer.

In addition to early stage and advance stage, there are in between stages that are stage 2 and stage 3. At stage 2, the cancer may or may not be detectable through a physical examination or imaging tests and still has not spread outside of the prostate. Then, at stage 3, the cancer has now spread beyond the prostate and may spread to the nearby seminal vesicles. This might include some stage-4 prostate cancers. As with local stage prostate cancers (stage 1 or early stage), the 5-year survival rate is nearly 100%.

American Cancer Society (2016b) suggested that radical prostatectomy and radiation therapy (external beam or brachytherapy) may also be appropriate options to eradicated stage 2 cancer. Then, treatment options for stage 3 cancer may include external beam radiation plus hormone therapy or plus brachytherapy. Hormone therapy is less aggressive treatment for men with other medical problems and older. Hormonal therapy uses drugs to block or lower testosterone and other male sex hormones that fuel cancer. This can stop or slow growth and spread of cancer.

References

American Cancer Society. (2016b). Initial treatment of prostate cancer, by stage. Retrieved from http://www.cancer.org/cancer/prostatecancer/detailedguide/prostate-cancer-treating-by-stage

Garnick, MB. (2016). Early-stage prostate cancer: Treat or wait? Harvard Medical School, Health Publications. Retrieved from http://www.harvardprostateknowledge.org/early-stage-prostate-cancer-treat-or-wait

Johansson JE., Andrén, O., Andersson, SO., Dickman, PW., Holmberg, L., Magnuson, A., and Adami, HO. (2004). Natural History of Early, Localized Prostate Cancer. The Journal of American Medical Association. Vol 291, No. 22. Retrieved from http://jama.jamanetwork.com/article.aspx?articleid=198897

Mayo Clinic Staff. (2014). Stage 4 prostate cancer. Mayo Clinic. Retrieved from http://www.mayoclinic.org/diseases-conditions/stage-4-prostate-cancer/basics/definition/con-20094020

09- Where is Starting Point of Testicular Cancer?

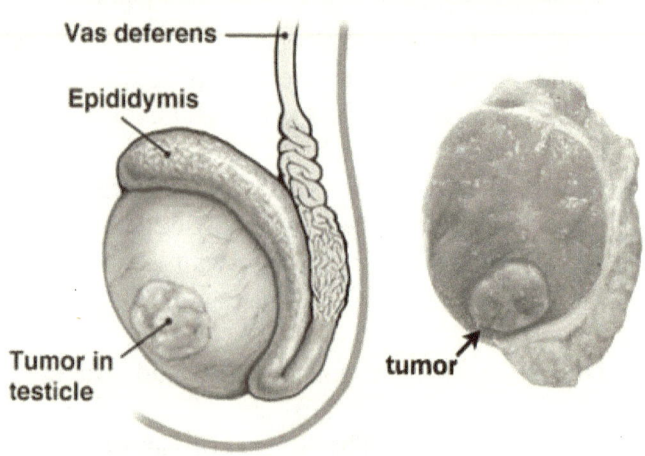

Testicular cancer (https://hudsonvalleypress.com)

    Organ called a testicle is another name for a testis which kinds of two small golf size organs are hanging under penis. The testis produces hormones such as testosterone and steroid. Testosterone is a male hormone, important to develop secondary sex attributes. Steroid hormones to manage our growth and development.

    Another crucial function of testis is to manufacture sperm, about 300 million sperm cells (equal to 5 milliliter) are produced each day. These sperm are used to fertilize a woman egg. One sperm needed only to fertilize an egg, other millions are dead during ejaculation.

It is not clear what cause testicular cancer, but we know that germ cells, sperm producers are starting point of cancer in testicles. The cells in the testicle are out of control, then changed from healthy to be called as tumor. The tumor could spread even to other tissues of body system.

Several risk factors of this cancer are "an undescended testicle, family history of testicular cancer, HIV infection, carcinoma in situ of the testicle, having had testicular cancer before, being of a certain race or ethnicity and body size" (American Cancer Society, 2018).

In addition to HIV (AIDS) infection, other viruses such as hepatitis C virus (HCV), Epstein-Barr virus (EBV) and Human papillomavirus (HPV) are believed to link to testicular cancer. In case of HPV, Garolla et al (2012) found infection of HPV on sperm of hundreds testis cancer patients. The infection negatively impacts on sperm motility and concentration during 12-month observations.

References
American Cancer Society. (2018, May 17). "Risk Factors for
      Testicular Cancer." Retrieved from
      https://www.cancer.org/cancer/testicular-cancer/causes-risks-prevention/risk-factors.html
Garolla, A., Pizzol, D., Bertoldo, A., Ghezzi, M., Carraro, U., Ferlin, A and Foresta, C. (2012, Dec 21). Testicular cancer and HPV semen infection. Front Endocrinol (Lausanne). 2012; 3: 172.

10- HPV Infects Nasal Cavity

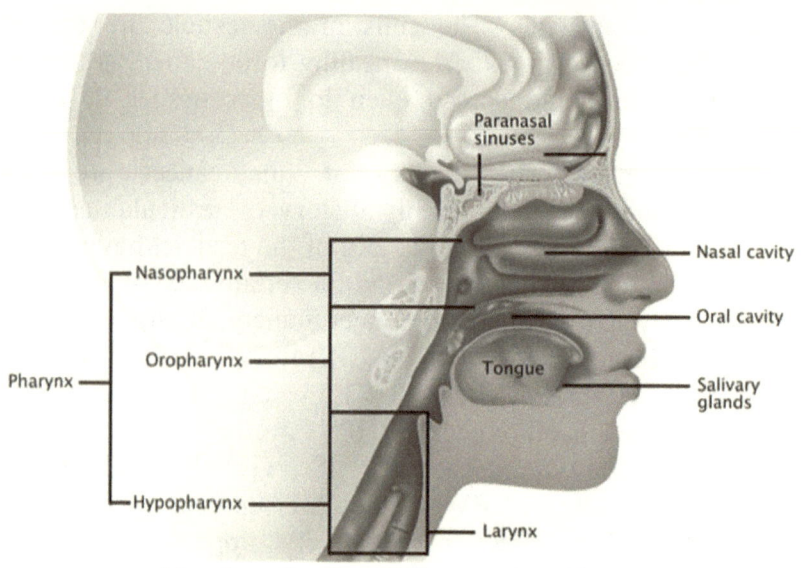

Nasal cavity (https://www.nhs.uk)

Virus types 6 and 11 are found in nasal cavity could produces some forms of tumors (papilloma) or warts. Infection likely ruins healthy tissues. These tumors or warts made a kind of bump, if big enough, the bump significantly alter sense of smell and decrease ability to breath.

Papilloma means fingerlike or nipplelike tumors grow outward, while inverted papilloma is tumor that grow inward to reach bone surface of nose.

HPV type 6 is less aggressive compared to HPV type 11, where type 11 migrates deep down into airway system, and causes sever infections. Even though very rarely, combination of pulmonary and esophageal lesions ends with mortality.

Tumors are not cancers, but so annoying. They grow from nose to the lung, disturb air passages in the respiratory tract. Growing tumor in larynx is commonly called as laryngeal papillomatosis. The Papilomas could be removed by small surgical operation but could grow back sometimes.

Incidents of nasal infection by HPV are estimated 20,000 cases per-year for both adult and children in the US. More severe to children than adult. Hoarseness and breathing difficulty are most common symptoms of nasal infections.

Children usually got infection from mother who infected with HPV during birth or in utero. The most incident occurs in group of children under 5 years old with symptoms of abnormal cry. Treatment is challenging, some children need surgery. In many cases, the infection is gone as children growing up.

11- Much More Americans Got Oral Infection by HPV Virus

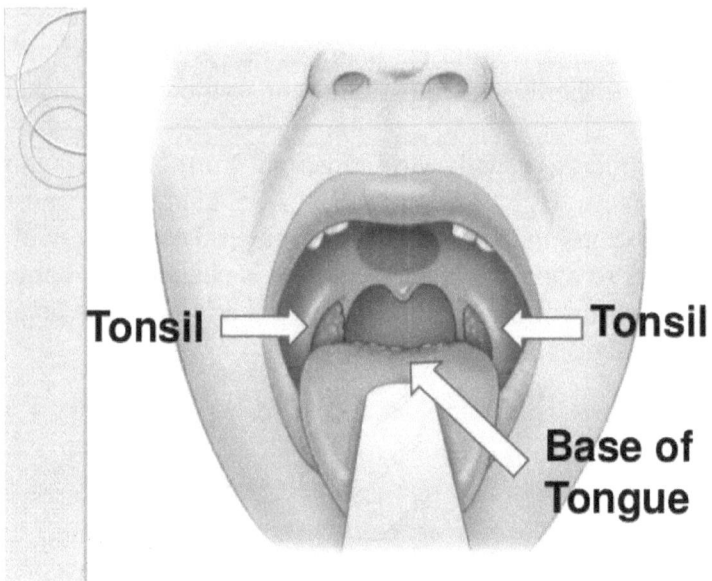

Oral infection by HVP (Miller, 2016)

Human papillomavirus incidence rate in oral is increasing in recent years. The viruses infect in the back of the mouth or throat. They are also colonizing in the tonsils and tongue base.

At least 14.2 million American got oral infection by HVP, quite surprisingly that men are infected more than women. Comparatively: 11 million men, while 3.2 million women infected to HPV only.

The estimate is alarming for near future, where 85% of population in the USA (and worldwide) will encounter oral Human Papillomavirus in some degree.

Risk factor of HPV infection is the men who had more than 20 sexual partners. High rate infections found in men who have sex with men. Men have genital infection with HPV tend to have oral infection too.

Cigarette and marijuana are risk factors as well. 10% greater risk for smokers who smokes more than 16 cigarettes a day, and 6% for marijuana users. Older men and women, above 50 years old are riskier compared to young populations.

There many possibilities why men infected more than women, one of them is women developed resistance in their immune system better than men. Thus, many women could rid of the HPV naturally from their mouth.

Unluckily, both men and women whose immune system compromises to HPV could develop oral cancer later in their life (take 20 years long from first infection). HPV type 16 mainly responsible to oral cancer. We will discuss oral cancer in the coming article.

Reference

Miller, RJ. 2016. Hpv virus infections and oropharynx cancer. Retrieved from https://www.slideshare.net/doctorbobm/hpv-virus-infections-and-oropharynx-cancer

12-Vaccine for Type 16 and 18 Viruses

HPV vaccine options

Vaccine	Who is it for?	How many doses?	What infections does it prevent?
Cervarix	Girls 9 to 26 years of age.	3	HPV types 16 and 18 (which cause cancer).
Gardasil	Girls and boys 9 to 26 years of age.	3	HPV types 6, 11 (which cause genital warts), and HPV 16 and 18 (which cause cancer).
Gardasil 9	Girls ages 9 to 26; boys ages 9 to 15.	3	HPV types 16, 18, 31, 33, 45, 52 and 58 (which cause cancer), and HPV types 6 or 11 (which cause warts).

Vaccines for penile and cervical cancers
(https://www.vox.com)

HPV vaccines are available in the market to protect human against many viruses, include virus types 6, 11, 16 and 18. As of previous article, types 6 and 11 responsible for genital's wart (please read previous article: HPV on Genitals Infection).

The types 16 and 18 of HPV viruses are highly believed to cause both men's penile cancer and women's cervical cancer.

Three vaccines are approved by the FDA to prevent HPV infection, and could be found in the market, they are Gardasil, Gardasil 9, and Cervarix. All three vaccines prevent infections with HPV types 6, 11, 16 and 18.

These vaccines are proven to reduce infections of genital and relate lesions both for women and men in the US. Vaccine doses for each girl and boy are presented at above Table.

Cervarix is used specially to prevent cervical cancer, and given to girls as early as 9 to 26 years of age. This vaccine need to be given 3 times at 0, 1 and 6 months period. Vaccine is effective to protect women from type 16 and 18 viruses.

Gardasil could be used by both boys and girls. The range of age and number of shots are the same with Cervarix vaccine. Period of shots at 0, 2 and 6 months, slightly different to Cervarix vaccine.

Gardasil 9 vaccine covers wide range of virus types. The vaccines could secure men and women from infection of virus types 6, 11, 16, 19, 31, 33, 45, 52 and 58. Administration of vaccine is 3 times shot with 0, 2 and 6 months period. Good for girls at 9 to 26 years old, and for boys at 15 to 26 years old.

13- Oral Cancer and HPV

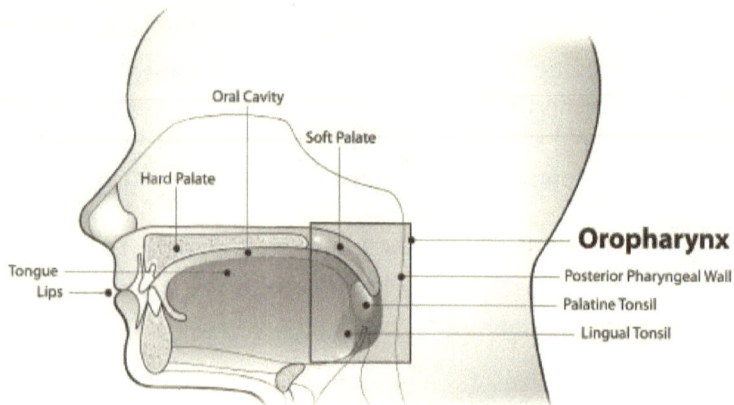

Oral cavity (https://www.cdc.gov)

We discussed the infection of oral due to virus at previous article (Much More American Got Oral Infection by Virus). If body can't get rid of virus or immune system is weak, virus may develop normal cells to be cancerous cells.

Some of oral cancer clear symptoms are swelling in mouth, color change of mouth tissue (a black or red), painful to swallowing and chewing in long time, mouth bleeding for more than 2 weeks, hoarse voice and sore throat persistently.

Like other cancer, it is long time to get cancer from first infection. Some studies showed that about 15 years to develop from virus infection to oral cancer.

HPV type 16 is found in oral to about 7% of US population. Of this, 1% of people is diagnosed with oral cancer. In term of number, 40 thousand people diagnosed with oral cancer in 2014 (WebMD, 2018). Women much less have oral cancer than men. Three times more men than women.

Whose oral is infected with virus, 32 time more likely to have cancer. Other risk factor is smoking and drinking. Smoker is 3 times risker than nonsmokers. Alcohol drinking will have 2.5 times likely to get oral cancer. It is fact that 75% people with oral cancer are smoking and drinking.

Survival rate is 80% for 1 year after diagnosed. The rate to be lower to 60% after 5 years diagnosed. The survival rate is lower compared to cervical cancer. 68% survival rate for cervical cancer after 5 years diagnosed.

Reference

WebMD. 2018. Oral Cancer. Retrieved from
    https://www.webmd.com/oral-health/guide/oral-cancer#1

14-HPV types 33 and 45

Common HPV Types and their effects

	HPV Types	Lead to:
Low-Risk	40, 42, 43, 44, 54, 61, 70, 72, 81	Benign cervical changes Genital warts
High-Risk	31, 33, 35, 39, 45, 51, 52, 56, 58, 59, 68, 73, 82	Precancer cervical changes Cervical cancer Anal and other cancers

1. Cox. *Baillère's Clin Obstet Gynaecol.* 1995;9:1.
2. Munoz et al. *N Engl J Med.* 2003;348:518.

Illustration (https://www.slideshare.net)

We knew that HPV types 16 and 18 caused cervical cancer (please read previous article: HPV Causes Cervical Cancer), and in addition that type 31 and 33 are also responsible to cervical cancer.

HPV type 33 is similar to type 16 in respect to its phylogenetically. In case of infections, HPV type 33 ranks fourth compare to other virus's types in the Northern America. The rank is following:
1. Type 16
2. Type 18
3. Type 45
4. Type 33

Based on study by Khouadri *et al* (2006) that of 5344 participants from several ethnicities and countries, that 89 patients (1.7%) contain HPV DNA type 33 in their cervical specimen. The degree of infections is from healthy (normal) to high grade infection of cervical cells.

HPV DNA type 45 was detected in 5% of 292 patients aged between 36 to 64 years old (Luiza et at, 2017). In addition to type 45, the study also found HPV DNA type HPV16, 18, 33-58 and HPV type 31.

It is believed that patients infected with multiple HVP types are more vulnerable and have lower survival rate after 5 years compared to patients who infected with single HPV type.

References

Khouadri, S., Villa, LL., Gagnon, S., Koushik, A., Richardson, H., Ferreira, S., Tellier, P., Simao, J., Matlashewski, G., Roger, M., Franco, EL., and Coutlée, F. 2006. Human Papillomavirus Type 33 Polymorphisms and High-Grade Squamous Intraepithelial Lesions of the Uterine Cervix. The Journal of Infectious Diseases, Volume 194, Issue 7, 1 October 2006, Pages 886–894.

Luiza, M et al. 2017. Multiple HPV genotype infection impact on invasive cervical cancer presentation and survival. Retrieved from http://journals.plos.org/plosone/article?id=10.1371/journal.pone.0182854

15- Anal Cancers and HPV

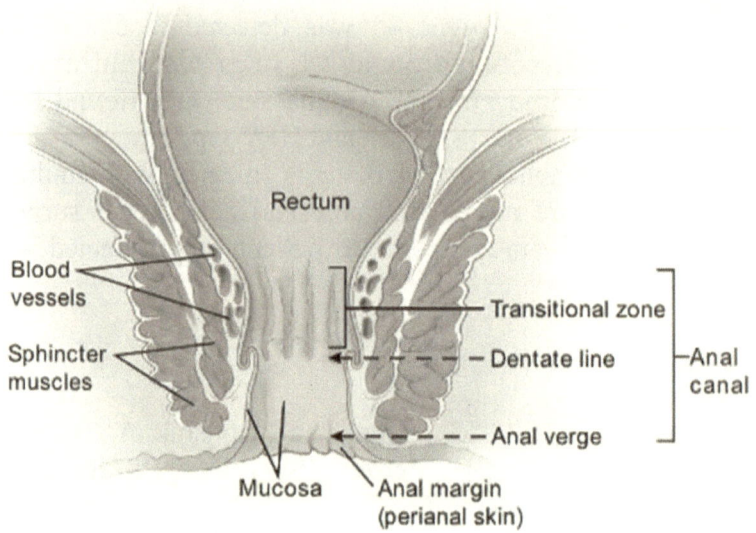

Anal canal and anus (https://www.cancer.org)

The infection by HPV may start cancer in anus, the infection is usually a sexually transmitted. HPV causes the cell grows out of control, then the infected normal cells were transformed into cancerous cells.

It is difficult to determine from where anal cancer starts, but many believed that anus cancer usually start from cells in mucosa. Cancers occupy in two parts: the anal canal and the anal margin.

The anal cancer is the same human papillomavirus (HPV) which caused on women cancer (cervical cancer). It is surprisingly that women who have cervical cancer will have higher probability to be infected by anal cancer virus.

HPV type 16 caused both cervix and anal cancers. HPV type 18 responsible to cervix, not anal cancer (please read previous article: Viruses Causes Cervical Cancer). Moreover, HPV type 6 and 11 cause anal and genital warts.

As reported by American Cancer Society (2017) that several risk factors of anal cancer are sexual activity, smoking, lower immunity, gender and age. In respect to gender and age that women are more common than men, and women with age more than 60 is higher risk than younger ones.

Reference

American Cancer Society. (2017, November 13). " Risk Factors for Anal Cancer." Retrieved from https://www.cancer.org/cancer/anal-cancer/causes-risks-prevention/risk-factors.html

16- Identification of Microorganism in Healthcare

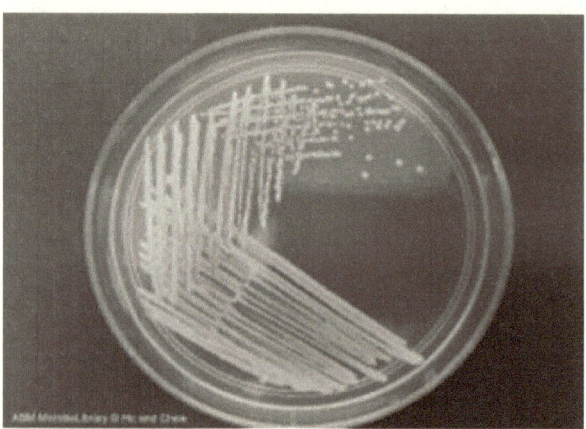

Staphylococcus aureus caused bone and joint infections

Virus is a microorganism, could be found easily in many kinds of environments: air, water or liquid, land and attaches to living creatures. This article is to give an idea how the procedure to identify microorganisms that important in healthcare and public health.

Although rapid microbial detection and molecular assays can be used to identify microorganism, growing and characterizing microorganism are still very important procedures used in clinical labs. Knowledge of selective or differential media and biochemical tests gained are used for diagnostic tests further on.

As an example, a doctor treating a patient with joint pain may subject blood samples to biochemical tests to determine the cause of inflammation. Bacteria known to cause bone (osteomyelitis) and joint (septic arthritis) infections include *Staphylococcus aureus, Enterobacter* species, and *Streptococcus* species.

Another example of how identification skills utilized are important in human medicine is the food poisoning epidemic of 2011. Over 2,000 German citizens were exposed to an unknown strain of *Escherichia coli*, over 600 of which developed haemolytic-uremic syndrome, a potentially fatal disease of the kidneys and nervous system.

Investigations by Germany health officials included streaking for isolation, Gram stains, biochemical tests, and culturing specimen on specialized, enriched culture media. They eventually discovered a new strain of *E.coli* now known as Enterohemorrhagic *E. coli* (EHEC, Figure at below)

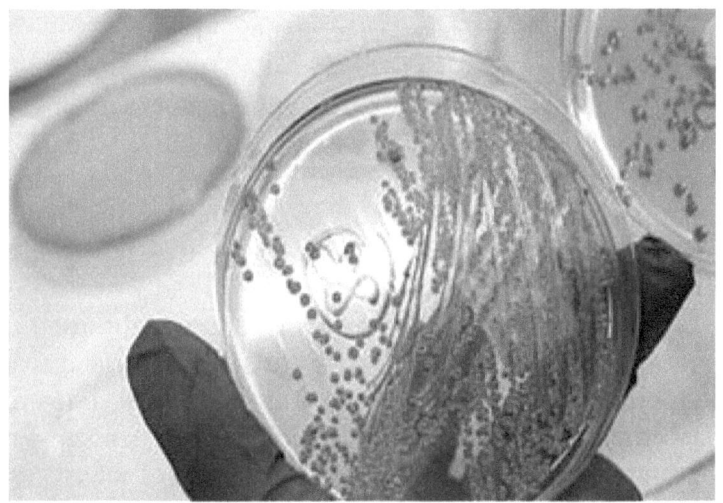

Enterohemorrhagic Escherichia coli

Thus, it is crucial to know what kinds of microorganism to cause what diseases, then the doctor could treat the diseases which caused by specific microorganism. Specific drug could be used to target specific microorganism.

17- Important of Microorganisms in Food Industry

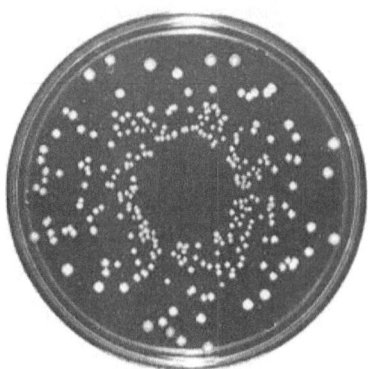

Lactobacillus casei, Shirota is used for enumeration of Bifidobacterial in fermented milks.

Our life might not exist without microorganisms, since these "tiny" unseen creatures help human being in many ways. They are digesting our food, fixing gases, decomposing waste and involving in may cycles like to break down dead organisms then to be used as fertilizer by living organism as part of food chain.

In industry, microorganisms are widely used in many industries, from small to large scale ones, and from traditional to cutting edge technology industries. Bacteria, yeast, molds, combination of several microorganisms and even virus are commonly used in many types of industries.

The types of industry include food industry (industrial products), pharmaceutical industry, biotech industry, agriculture industry and waste treatment (reduce toxic pollutants).

In food processing, our ancestors routinely used microorganisms for production of beverages, sausages and dairy products. Currently, we could use microorganisms of naturally occurring and genetically modified microorganism to increase food production.

These products (beverages, sausages and dairy products) could be improved their health benefit to public by attaching probiotic microorganisms. The health benefits include to improve digestion, to protect body from pathogens, increase peristaltic activity in intestine and stimulate immune system.

Above figure (top of this article) shown an example of probiotic microbes from lactic acid bacteria group. The bacteria called Lactobacillus casei, Shirota is used in dairy product to improve nutritional and health benefit. The Japan company, Honsha used this bacterium to produce Yakult. The Yakult is believed nutrient rich drink and could improve immune system.

18- Virus that Kill Cancer

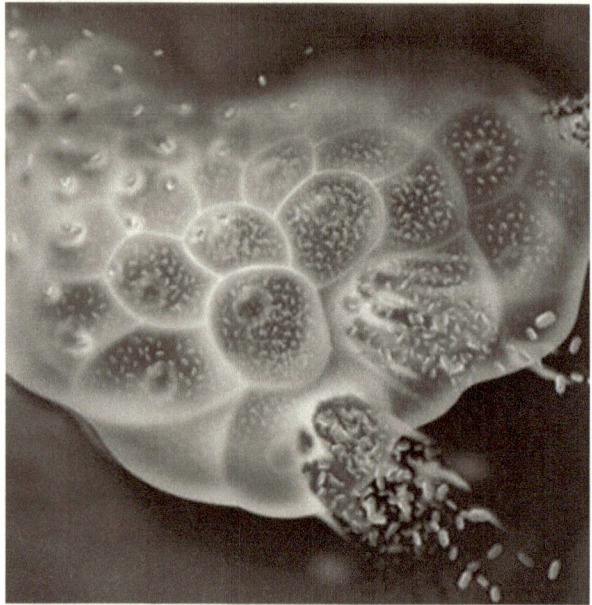

Virus attacked cancer cells (http://healthdoctrine.com)

Many researchers tried to find out radical treatments to control cancer cells. It is because "traditional ways" is insufficient to cure patients that growing in highly number in recent years. One in every three of persons will get and dying due to cancer in the North America.

Long time treatment through surgery removal or radiation is not sufficient to cure patients with some specific cancers, and even the cancer cells keep growing faster after treatments. Then, the Ottawa Hospital Research Institute in Canada started to use "advance method" by using virus to kill cancer cells. The research finding is amazing that virus selected the cancer cells only, ignore the healthy ones.

Scientists successfully using measles virus to control brain tumor that infected patients in the Illinois,

USA. Virus was "inserted" by specific gene to recognize protein in the cancer cells, thus not destroy non-infected cells.

Other promising research showed that measles virus type delta 24 could stop tumor growing in the mice. A chosen volunteer feel optimism with this kind of treatments, after uncertainty with chemo and radiation treatments for quite longer periods.

Surprisingly, scientists move further by using engineered HIV virus to cure leukemia. Patient feel healthier with no more fevers and comma after treatments.

This kind of approach to deal with cancer cells is at early stages. No guarantee to success to cure to all type of cancers, but on-going works could make possible to control cancer cells in the near future.

19- Perplexing between HIV and HPV

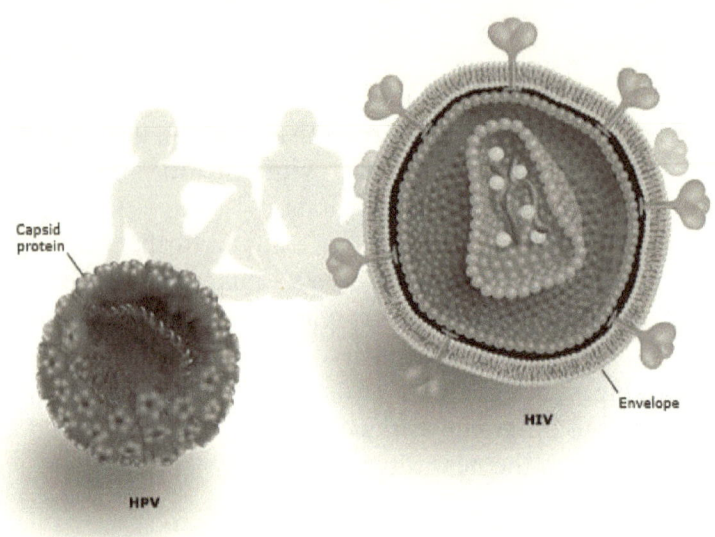

Different of HPV and HIV
(Credit to: Brandon Brown *et al*, 2013)

If you don't know the different between Human immunodeficiency virus (HIV) and Human papillomavirus (HPV), don't be worry, you are not only one who confuses. As reported by NBC News on May 28, 2018 that president Donald Trump asked Bill Gates to explain the different between HPV and HIV.

In term of target, HPV infects moist membranes and skin, while HIV infects immune system. Infection through sexual transmission is common for both virus, and cause health problems worldwide.

HPV develops diseases called as genital warts, verruca and even cancers. More than 79 million Americans of early 20's affected by this virus. Luckily, vaccines are developed to prevent the spreading of HPV.

In case HIV attacked immune system, the virus will destroy cells to fight diseases, then develop to Acquired Immune Deficiency Syndrome (AIDS). Development to AIDS could be halted if early diagnosed.

Antiretrovirals Therapy (ART) is designed to block progressive development of HIV. The ART not kill virus not cure AID, its just to slow down the process of weakening immune system and virus replicating.

There are more than 30 kinds of drugs for HIV infection and much more supplements available in the markets. These drugs have been approved by Food and Drug Administration (FDA), but must be used under doctor recommendations.

Patients usually eat two combination drugs, and never miss. Absence from taking medication for a while will promote HIV to develop new strain that drug resistance. Even drugs can not cure the infection, However, ART may improve patient's quality of life, and no transmission of virus to other people.

About the Author

Evi Erlinda graduated from department of Biology Human Medicine at Franciscan University. USA. Pursued internship at Earl K Hospital and Our Lady of the Lake Hospital, both in the USA. Experienced to teach Microbiology at under graduate level.

www.ingramcontent.com/pod-product-compliance
Lightning Source LLC
Chambersburg PA
CBHW030517220526
45464CB00006B/2834